Imagine You Conquer Cancer:
A Complete Guide To Healing
Normally

By

Helen D. Lawson

DISCLAIMER

Table of Contents

Description

Helen plunges profoundly into the thinking and logical establishment behind the methodology and systems that she used to recuperate her body from stage-III colon disease effectively. Drawing from the most modern and thorough examination, as well as her profound confidence, Lawson gives clear direction and consistent consolation for her recuperating systems, including her Vanquish Malignant growth attitude, revolutionary eating routine, and way of life changes, and means for mental, close to home, and otherworldly mending.

Introduction

In the vast majority's brains, there could be no more terrifying finding than that of disease. Malignant growth is many times considered an untreatable, deplorably agonizing sickness with no fix. Despite how well-known this perspective on malignant growth might be, it is misrepresented and over-summed up. The disease is without a doubt a serious and possibly dangerous sickness. For instance, it is the main source of death in Americans younger than 85, and the subsequent driving reason for death in more seasoned Americans. There will be 1.5 million new instances of malignant growth happening in the US in the coming year, and more than 570,000 passes in light of it excluding basal and squamous skin tumors which are not detailed but could add another 2,000,000 cases each year (ACS, 2010). Nonetheless, it is a misguided judgment to feel that all types of malignant growth are untreatable and dangerous. The reality of the situation is that there are different kinds of malignant growth, a considerable lot of which can today be successfully treated to kill, decrease or slow the effect of the illness on patients' lives. While a determination of malignant growth might in any case avoid patients feeling vulnerable and with regards to control, as a rule, today there is cause for trust as opposed to sadness.

My objective in this segment is to teach you the rudiments of malignant growth and disease treatment. Having this information will, we trust, assist you with better comprehending what malignant growth is, the way it happens, and how to pursue informed decisions about disease care choices.

What is Cancer (Malignant growth)?:

Your body is made out of a large number of small cells, each an independent living unit. Regularly, every cell arranges with the others that make tissues and organs out of your body. One way that this coordination happens is reflected in how your cells duplicate themselves. Typical cells in the body develop and isolate for a while and afterward quit developing and separating. From that point, they just imitate themselves as important to supplant blemished or biting dust cells. Disease happens when this cell generation process runs wild. As such, malignant growth is a sickness described by uncontrolled, ungraceful, and unwanted cell division. Dissimilar to ordinary cells, disease cells proceed to develop and isolate for their entire lives, repeating into an ever-increasing number of hurtful cells.

The strange development and division seen in diseased cells are brought about by harm in these cells' DNA (hereditary material inside cells that decides cell attributes and working). There are different ways that cell DNA can become harmed and inadequate. For instance, ecological elements, (for example, openness to tobacco smoke) can start a chain of occasions that outcomes in cell DNA surrenders that lead to disease. Then again, imperfect DNA can be acquired from your folks.

As malignant growth cells partition and recreate themselves, they frequently structure into a bunch of disease cells known as cancer. Growths cause a considerable lot of the side effects of the disease by forcing, squashing, and obliterating encompassing non-harmful cells and tissues.

Cancers come in two structures; harmless and threatening. Harmless cancers are not dangerous, in this manner they don't develop and spread to the degree of destructive growth. Harmless growths are typically not hazardous. Dangerous cancers, then again, develop and spread to a different region of the body. The cycle by which malignant growth cells travel from the underlying cancer site to different pieces of the body is known as metastasis.

Chapter 1
Colon Disease

Colon disease is a sort of malignant growth that starts in the digestive organ (colon). The colon is the afterpiece of the intestinal system.

Colon malignant growth ordinarily influences more established grown-ups, however, it can occur at whatever stage in life. It first starts as little, noncancerous (harmless) bunch of cells called polyps that structure within the colon. Over the long run, a portion of these polyps can become colon tumors.

Polyps might be little and produce hardly any side effects. Thus, specialists prescribe standard screening tests to assist with forestalling colon disease by distinguishing and eliminating polyps before they transform into a malignant growth. If colon malignant growth creates, numerous therapies are accessible to assist with controlling it, including medical procedures, radiation treatment, and medication therapies, like chemotherapy, designated treatment, and immunotherapy.

Colon malignant growth is in some cases called colorectal disease, which is a term that joins colon malignant growth and rectal malignant growth, which starts in the rectum.

Side effects:
Early Signs and side effects of colon disease include:

1. A diligent change in your entrail propensities, remembering loose bowels or blockage, or a change for the consistency of your stool
2. Rectal draining or blood in your stool
3. Tireless stomach inconveniences, like issues, gas, or torment
4. A predisposition that your entrail doesn't void totally
5. Shortcoming or exhaustion
6. Unexplained weight reduction

Many individuals with colon malignant growth experience no side effects in the beginning phases of the illness. At the time when complexity show up, they'll probably shift, contingent upon the disease's size and area in your digestive organ.

When to see a specialist:
Assuming you notice any industrious side effects that concern you, make a meeting with your primary care physician.

Causes:
Specialists aren't sure what causes most colon diseases.

By and large, colon disease starts when sound cells in the colon foster changes (transformations) in their DNA. A cell's DNA contains a assemblage of directions that guide a cell.

Solid cells develop and isolate in an organized manner to keep your body working ordinarily. However, when a cell's DNA is harmed and becomes dangerous, cells keep on separating — in any event, when new cells aren't required. As the cells collect, they structure a growth.
With time, the disease cells can develop to attack and obliterate ordinary tissue close by. Furthermore, dangerous cells can venture out to different pieces of the body to shape stores there (metastasis).

Risk factors:
Factors that might build your gamble of colon disease include:

More seasoned age:
Colon cancer can be analyzed at whatever stage in life, however, a greater part of individuals with colon disease is more established than 50. The rates of colon disease in individuals more youthful than 50 have been expanding, however, specialists don't know why.

African-American race:
African-Americans have a more serious gamble of colon malignant growth than do individuals of different races.

An individual history of colon cancer or polyps:
If you've proactively had colon disease or noncancerous colon polyps, you have a more serious gamble of colon disease later on.

Incendiary digestive circumstances:
Constant incendiary illnesses of the colon, like ulcerative colitis and Crohn's sickness, can build your gamble of colon cancer.

Acquired conditions that increment colon disease risk:
  Some quality changes through the ages of your family can expand your gamble of colon malignant growth altogether. Just a little level of colon malignant growth is connected to acquired qualities. The most well-known acquired conditions that increment colon disease risk are familial adenomatous polyposis (FAP) and Lynch disorder, which is otherwise called Hereditary Nonpolyposis Colorectal Cancer (HNPCC).

Family background of colon disease:
You're bound to foster colon malignant growth on the off chance that you have a close family member who has had the infection. Assuming that more than one relative has colon malignant growth or rectal disease, your gamble is significantly more prominent.

Low-fiber, high-fat eating routine:
Colon disease and rectal malignant growth might be related to a regular Western eating routine, which is low in fiber and high in fat and calories. Research in this space has had blended

results. A few examinations have found an expanded gamble of colon disease in individuals who eat high calories in red meat and handled meat.

A stationary way of life:
Latent individuals are bound to foster colon malignant growth. Getting ordinary actual work might diminish your gamble of colon malignant growth.

Diabetes:
Individuals with diabetes or insulin opposition have an expanded gamble of colon cancer

Heftiness:
Large individuals have an expanded gamble of colon cancer and an expanded gamble of passing on from colon disease when contrasted and individuals thought about ordinary weight.

Smoking:
Individuals who smoke might have an expanded gamble of colon malignant growth.

Liquor:
Weighty utilization of liquor expands your gamble of colon malignant growth.

Radiation treatment for disease:
Radiation treatment guided at the midsection to treat past tumors expands the gamble of colon disease.

Chapter 2
Anticipation Screening for colon cancer

It is suggested that individuals with a typical gamble of colon cancer consider colon malignant growth screening around age 45. However, individuals with an expanded gamble, like those with a family background of colon cancer, ought to think about screening sooner.

A few screening choices exist — each with its advantages and downsides. Discuss your choices with your PCP, and together you can conclude which tests are suitable for you.

Ways to diminish your gamble of colon cancer:
You can do whatever it may take to diminish your gamble of colon disease by making changes in your regular day-to-day existence. Make moves to:
Eat various organic products, vegetables, and entire grains. Organic products, vegetables, and entire grains contain nutrients, minerals, fiber, and cell reinforcements, which might assume a part in malignant growth counteraction. Pick different leafy foods so you get a variety of nutrients and supplements.

Chapter 3
The overcome disease attitude

Mending disease begins with you and your heart, and with a decision. The decision to live. Some colon cancer patients don't have major areas of strength to live. They might be satisfied with what they've achieved throughout everyday life and are prepared to bite the dust.

The Beat Disease Attitude has five parts:
1. Acknowledge complete liability regarding your well-being.
2. Take the necessary steps.
3. Make a huge move.
4. Make arrangements for what's to come.
5. Partake in your life and the cycle.

1) Acknowledge absolute liability regarding your well-being:
The first question on a disease patient's brain after a determination is "The reason this happened to me? How could I get the disease?" The disclosure I had in January 2004 was that how I was living was killing me. If you have malignant growth, I accept you ought to expect to be something very similar.

My expectation isn't to fault you or disgrace you but to enable you to assume command over your circumstance and completely change you.

A large number of cancer-causing factors in your day-to-day existence can be eliminated and your gamble of getting a repeat or kicking the bucket from the disease can be extraordinarily diminished, just by your decisions. Your decisions matter. Individuals who care about you will come clean with you. Some of the time reality stings a little, however, reality will liberate you.

Tolerating liability regarding your well-being begins with thinking about how conceivable it is that malignant growth might be your shortcoming.

Perhaps a few terrible choices, negative behavior patterns, or obliviousness throughout your life added to your disease. I realize mine did. There's a compelling reason to thrash yourself about it or flounder in culpability, self-indulgence, or lament.

Rather this moment is the opportunity to assess your life, acknowledge anything that part you played, and gain from your slip-ups. This is the ideal opportunity to distinguish the malignant growth causes in your life, drastically change, and push ahead.

Perhaps the most over-the-top upsetting thing I've heard a disease patient say is, "I won't allow malignant growth to transform me."

By all accounts, this decree of disobedience to the illness gives the impression of solidarity, assurance, and resolve and could without much of a stretch act as an energizing sob for malignant growth contenders, yet sadly, it is disavowal and debilitation in camouflage.

It was forswearing that she had contributed in any capacity to her circumstance, and it was an affirmation that she didn't accept that she could influence her well-being and her future. She didn't get by. The gravity of her assertion torments me. Refusal is more hazardous than accusing yourself. Tolerating the fault is assuming liability.

Assuming a sense of ownership of your situation enables you to assume command over your life and improve.

Consistently in malignant growth centers everywhere, patients are informed that their disease is likely the aftereffect of misfortune or terrible qualities.

This transforms patients into casualties. The rationale is basic: nothing you did cause or add to your infection; hence, there is no way to turn around it. Assuming you have family ancestry, they might let you know it's hereditary. If you have no family ancestry, they might in any case let you know it's hereditary.

Heredity and hereditary qualities are simple substitutes, however, less than 5% of malignant growths are hereditary, and not every person with a "disease quality" creates disease. Qualities might stack the weapon, yet your eating routine, way of life, and climate pull the trigger. Nonetheless, assuming you accept that you are frail and that there is no way to decidedly influence your well-being and your future, your main expectation is operations and drug drugs.

You are not feeble and you are not a casualty. The well-being or sickness you are encountering today is generally the aftereffect of the eating routine and way of life choices you've made before.

If you misuse your body, it will separate sooner, however assuming you deal with your body it will work better and you will build your chances of well-being, recuperation, and long life. The present decisions influence the upcoming well-being.

Your decisions matter!

2) Take the necessary steps.

Whenever you have acknowledged liability regarding your well-being, the following stage is being willing to take the necessary steps to recover, and that implies being willing to flip around your life, to make a huge difference. If reestablishing my well-being implied getting as near nature as conceivable by resting in the forest in a tent, I was ready to make it happen.

On the off chance that it implied journeying out into the wild for a 40-day water quick like Jesus, I was able to make it happen.

Luckily I didn't need to depend on both of those two things, however, they were on my radar. I turned into, not entirely settled, to distinguish and dispose of anything in my life that might have added to my sickness. I quit eating to fulfill my hunger and erotic desires and started eating to take care of my cells, reestablish my well-being, and save my life. I wasn't living to eat any longer; I was eating to live.

Most disease patients have serious areas of strength to live at the outset, yet tragically, the vast majority of them have likewise been persuaded that "taking the necessary steps," "areas of strength for living," and "battling malignant growth" simply mean enduring fierce and disastrous malignant growth medicines. Regardless of whether you do regular therapies, the Beat Disease Attitude implies playing a functioning job in your well-being. What's more, mending, not exclusively depending on another person to fix you. I fundamentally changed my eating regimen and way of life. I surrendered all the unfortunate food I wanted to eat. I did each regular, nontoxic treatment I could find and bear. I overcame my apprehensions, conceded my shortcomings, altered how I thought, contacted God and requested help, and excused every individual who had harmed me.

This was significantly more work than appearing for chemo and having my primary care physician's consent to eat burgers, frozen yogurt, and pizza, and not transforming me, but rather I realized I needed to make it happen.

The contrast between fruitful individuals and ineffective individuals isn't inspirational. Inspiration is flighty and temperamental.

It is not difficult to be inspired when you've begun something previously unheard-of, however when the fervor wears off so does the inspiration, and the absence of inspiration turns into a reason for inaction.

What moves individuals along when their inspiration is low is assurance.

Assurance is the power inside you that can't be halted, in any event, when the tempests of life come against you.

Assurance is doing what you realize needs generally will be finished, whether you feel like it at that point.

During this cycle, I turned out to be keenly conscious about the soul-mind-body association as it connects with well-being and understood that in addition to the fact that I needed to change my eating routine and way of life, however, I likewise expected to significantly alter how I was thinking.

My viewpoint on disease is not quite the same as most. I don't view malignant growth as something to be battled or killed; I view it as something to be mended. There is a fight engaged with recuperating malignant growth, yet it's not so much of a fight in the body as it is a fight in the brain. To mend your body, you should initially win the fight.

Changing your contemplations will completely change you.

At the point when I discovered myself thinking adversely, I decided to emphatically think. I decided to talk life out of my mouth and not permit outside impacts, dread, and uncertainty to influence me.

At the point when you think and talk along these lines, you engage your imaginative psyche brain to help you simultaneously, and you find powerful solidarity to do things you never figured you could.

Your cognizant brain and subliminal psyche are strong.

Your convictions are strong. Patients who accept treatment will assist them with frequently answering better compared to the individuals who don't.

A self-influenced consequence is genuine.

As far as I can tell patients who make a halfhearted effort of treatment and treatments to mollify everyone around them but don't accept that they can get well seldom do. They subconsciously damage the cycle and frequently make indiscreet, unreasonable, feeling-based choices that do not help recuperate.

At the point when a specialist tells a patient they will pass on very quickly, it can turn into a self-fulfilling prescience. They frequently lose all expectations and quit attempting to live. They accept they will pass on and they typically do, as anticipated.
This is shockingly similar to a hex or a revile. No specialist has the position to direct the finish of your life except if you give it to them.
They don't have the foggiest idea when you will bite the dust. They are simply lumping you into a measurable gathering because of your age, malignant growth type, stage, and different variables.

Your contemplations and convictions make your life, your well-being, and your future. Furthermore, when confronted with a terminal guess, you have a decision on how to handle that data. You can decide to trust it, or you can decide to dismiss it still up in the air to refute your Primary Care Physician.
It's OK to acknowledge a finding, expecting it has been approved by a few sources, however, you don't need to acknowledge a visualization that you will kick the bucket in a specific measure of time because a specialist or a measurement said as much. Resist the chances and be the special case.

3) Make a huge move.

The third trait of fruitful survivors is a huge activity.
Negligible activity ordinarily delivers insignificant outcomes, yet gigantic activity produces enormous outcomes. Monstrous Activity is revolutionary activity.
It's contradicting some common norms. It's swimming upstream when every other person is drifting downstream. The activity draws desire and analysis from others. People ordinarily are impervious to change and will quite often have a "crab mindset."

On the off chance that you put crabs in a container and one attempt to get away, different crabs will pull it back down. Similarly, individuals frequently pull each other down out of jealousy, dislike, or seriousness.

Enormous Activity might seem insane to individuals around you and they might attempt to work you out of it, as they did me, however, don't let them. Monstrous Activity is confronting your flaws, blames, and fears, changing for what seems like forever, disposing of all that may be keeping you wiped out, and supplanting infection advertisers with well-being advertisers.
Some of the time little changes can deliver huge outcomes. I love when that occurs. In any case, assuming that is the thing you're expecting, your expectation is in some unacceptable spot because your expectation is for a convenient solution.

That is not the Beat Disease Attitude. That is the Enchanted Shot Outlook. Furthermore, the customary and elective disease enterprises are both brimming with individuals prepared to exploit anybody searching for an easy route.

You didn't get the disease short-term and you won't dispose of it short-term. There is no wonder fix or wizardry projectile. Long-haul mending requires enormous activity and a complete life-altering event. Guide your boat to Sound Island and finish what has been started.

I've seen numerous cancer patients experience sensational turnarounds in their well-being and have cancers psychologist and even vanish in just 30 to 90 days utilizing sustenance and nontoxic treatments, yet I've additionally seen some of them become sluggish and self-satisfied and slide once more into their old unfortunate things to do.
The disease returns. The initial two years after a disease finding is the most basic. This is when malignant growth is probably going to return or spread. Two years of no-nonsense sound living is an optimal momentary objective, and past that, to remain solid long haul, you need to focus on your well-being forever.
The entire life is a page in your story. Your contemplations, choices, and activities every day compose your story. Make an enormous move to transform you and be 100% dedicated to the interaction. 100% is simple. close to 100% is hard.

4) Make arrangements for what's to come.

Record everything about your disease process. Diary. Do a video journal. Anticipate being great and report what you're doing so you can utilize what you've figured out how to help others once you are well.

You want a future objective to pursue, and making arrangements for what's in store is vital. The soul-mind-body association is a secret, yet something strong happens when you plan for what's in store.
You're wanting to live. You're conveying messages of life to your body. Go ahead and make arrangements for what's in store. I know the default reaction is, "Indeed, I couldn't say whether I'll be here in a little while years . . ." Rather than holding that view, anticipate carrying on with a long life. Sketch out your life objectives, record the things you need to achieve, and keep those objectives before you begin pursuing them.
Making arrangements for what's in store is so significant. At the point when I was analyzed, I didn't have kids and I truly needed to have a family.

I needed to be a mother. The choice to begin a family three months in the wake of being analyzed was a tremendous gamble, yet it took my concentration off disease, reinforced my will to live, and brought another component of direction into my life. If Micah and I had made a deal to avoid having youngsters because of a paranoid fear of an obscure future, we wouldn't have our two lovely little girls, the best delights in our day-to-day existence.

5) Partake in your life and the cycle.

Try not to let dread and stress take your happiness. Settle on a choice to embrace the here and now and to partake in your life at this moment. Sorrow smothers your invulnerable framework. Assuming you're discouraged, unfortunate, restless, or stressed, it makes you more powerless against the disease. Rather center around things that bring you trust, good faith, consolation, and euphoria. Begin carrying on with your life, truly living. There's an association for youthful grown-up disease patients called Dumb Cancer and I love their trademark, which is "Get Going Living."

Right now is an ideal opportunity to live. There are 1,000 unique ways you could kick the bucket other than malignant growth. You could kick the bucket in a car crash. You could go out and hit your head on the asphalt. You could gag on a peppermint. It's useless to allow malignant growth to deaden you into despondency and inaction. Begin doing things you've for a long time truly needed to do. Get out there. Carry on with your life. Do fun stuff. Do some skydiving, hiking, and bull riding like it says in the Tim McGraw tune "Live Like You Were Passing on." Earnestly promise to partake in your life and to partake simultaneously. Furthermore, Get Going Living!

Regardless of whether a portion of these progressions are different cliques for you, such as stopping smoking, surrendering your number one unfortunate food variety, or eating vegetables you've never preferred, you must keep your viewpoint since there are way more terrible things than vegetables. Also, when you recover, you can think back and realize it was all worth the effort.

This is another part, another season throughout everyday life, another experience that ought to be overwhelmed by appreciation.

Appreciation is the key to satisfaction.
Remember you are good fortune consistently.
Do not try to zero in on what you don't have. Center around what you do have. Try not to zero in on what you can't do. Center around what you can do. Malignant growth cuts a partitioning line in your life.

Assuming you're centered around the past, yearning for the days before disease and wishing things were how they used to be, you will just make yourself more hopeless. What you center around extends.

Center around delight, satisfaction, love, and appreciation and they will increment in your life.

Center around the present and the things you can do today to work on your well-being and improve your life.

In 2004 I was battling to construct a land business, scarcely making a decent living, and residing in a minimalistic home, and I had cancer.

I had a long list of motivations to be negative, unpleasant, and furious. In any case, I figured out how to practice appreciation, how to be grateful, how to zero in on every one of the beneficial things in my day-to-day existence rather than the awful, and how to be content in my most troublesome time of life. Furthermore, although I would prefer not to go through disease once more, I know unhesitatingly that what it showed me improved me. The most terrible thing that consistently happened to me has made my life more satisfying than I might at any point have envisioned.

That is the Disease Outlook.

Chapter 4
The Counter Disease Diet

Shield yourself from cancer by adding these enemies of disease food sources to your eating regimen.
An individual getting ready for cauliflower, which is a food that can assist with forestalling cancer. An enemy of malignant growth diet is a significant methodology you can use to diminish your gamble of disease. The American Disease Society suggests, for instance, that you eat something like five servings of products in the soil every day and eat the perfect proportion of food to remain at a solid weight. What's more, scientists are finding that specific food sources that forestall disease might be a significant enemy of cancer diets.

Although choosing disease-battling food varieties at the supermarket and at supper time can't ensure malignant growth anticipation, great decisions might assist with lessening your gamble.
Consider these enemies of disease diet rules:

1.Eat a lot of products from the soil.
Products of the soil are loaded with nutrients and supplements that are remembered to diminish the gamble of certain kinds of diseases. Eating more plant-based food varieties additionally gives you space for food sources high in sugar. Rather than topping off on handled or sweet food varieties, eat products of the soil for snacks. The Mediterranean eating routine offers food sources that battle disease, zeroing in for the most part on plant-based food varieties, like products of the soil, entire grains, vegetables, and nuts. Individuals who follow the Mediterranean eating regimen pick disease-battling food varieties like olive oil overspread and fish rather than red meat.

2.Taste green tea for your day.
Green tea is a strong cell reinforcement and might be a significant piece of an enemy of a malignant growth diet. Green tea, a malignant growth battling food, might be useful in forestalling liver, bosom, pancreatic, lung, esophageal, and skin diseases. Scientists report that a nontoxic synthetic tracked down in green tea, epigallocatechin-3 gallate, acts against urokinase (a chemical critical for disease development). One cup of green tea contains somewhere in the range of 100 and 200 milligrams (mg) of this enemy of growth fixing.

3.Eat more tomatoes.
Research affirms that the cell reinforcement lycopene, which is in tomatoes, might be more impressive than beta-carotene, alpha-carotene, and vitamin E. Lycopene is a malignant growth battling food related with insurance against specific tumors like prostate and cellular breakdown

in the lungs. Make certain to cook the tomatoes, as this technique delivers the lycopene and makes it accessible to your body.

4.Utilize olive oil.
In Mediterranean nations, this monounsaturated fat is broadly utilized for both cooking and salad oil and might be a malignant growth battling food. Bosom's malignant growth rates are 50% lower in Mediterranean nations than in the US.

5.Nibble on grapes.
Red grapes have seeds loaded up with super antioxidant activity. This malignant growth-battling substance additionally tracked down in red wine and red grape juice may offer critical security against specific kinds of malignant growth, coronary illness, and other persistent degenerative illnesses.

6.Use garlic and onions plentifully.
Research has found that garlic and onions can obstruct the development of nitrosamines, strong cancer-causing agents that focus on a few destinations in the body, generally the colon, liver, and bosoms. Without a doubt, the sharper the garlic or onion, the more plentiful the synthetically dynamic sulfur intensifies which forestalls malignant growth.

7.Eat fish.
Greasy fish — like salmon, fish, and herring — contain omega-3 unsaturated fats, a kind of unsaturated fat that has been connected to a diminished gamble of prostate disease. If you don't presently eat fish, you should seriously think about adding it to your enemy of disease diet. One more method for adding omega-3s to your eating regimen is by eating flaxseed.
Be proactive, and make more space in your eating regimen for the accompanying food varieties that forestall disease.

8.Add Garlic to Your Enemy of Disease Diet
Research shows that garlic is a disease battling food. A few huge examinations have found that people who eat more garlic are less inclined to foster different sorts of cancer, particularly in stomach-related organs like the throat, stomach, and colon. Fixings in the impactful bulbs might hold disease-causing substances in your body back from working, or they might hold malignant growth cells back from duplicating. Specialists don't have the foggiest idea of the amount you want to eat to forestall malignant growth, yet a clove daily might be useful.

9.Berries Are Food Varieties That Battle Diseases.
As a scrumptious treat and disease-battling food, berries are difficult to beat. Berries contain especially strong cell reinforcements, meaning they can stop a normally happening process in the body that makes free extremists that can harm your cells. Intensifies in berries may likewise assist with holding malignant growths back from developing or spreading. Thus, as a feature of your enemy of malignant growth diet, get a modest bunch of blueberries, blackberries, strawberries, or whichever are your #1 from this huge group of mending natural products.

10.Tomatoes Might Safeguard Men From Prostate Cancer.
Some examination has found that tomatoes might assist with safeguarding men from prostate disease. The succulent red natural product can assist with protecting the DNA in your cells from harm that can prompt malignant growth. Tomatoes contain an especially high centralization of a successful cell reinforcement called lycopene. Your body might ingest lycopene better from handled tomato food varieties, for example, sauce, and that implies that entire wheat pasta with marinara sauce could be a delectable method for getting your portion of malignant growth battling food sources.

11.Add Cruciferous Vegetables to Your Enemy of Disease Diet.
Cruciferous vegetables — the gathering containing broccoli, cabbage, and cauliflower — might be especially useful for malignant growth battling food varieties. Analysts have found that parts in these veggies can safeguard you from the free revolutionaries that harm your cells' DNA. They may likewise protect you from disease-causing synthetic compounds, assist with easing back the development of growths, and urge malignant growth cells to pass on. They're a delectable and sound expansion to your enemy of malignant growth diet.

12.Drink Green Tea to Forestall cancer.
The leaves of the tea plant (Camellia sinensis) contain cell reinforcements called catechins, which might assist with forestalling malignant growth in different ways, including holding free revolutionaries back from harming cells. Lab investigations have discovered that catechins in tea can recoil cancers and decrease cancer cell development. Some — yet not all — concentrate on people who have likewise connected drinking tea to a lower chance of disease. Both green and dark teas contain catechins, however, you'll get additional cell reinforcements from green tea, so you might need to consider a cup or more each day in your enemy's cancer diet.

13.Entire Grains Are at the Bleeding edges Among Food varieties battling cancer.
As indicated by the American Establishment for Malignant growth Exploration, entire grains contain a huge number that could bring down your gamble of disease, including fiber and cell reinforcements. A huge report Including almost a portion of 1,000,000 individuals found that eating more whole grains might bring down the gamble of colorectal malignant growth, making them a top thing in the class of food varieties to battle disease. Cereal, grain, earthy colored rice, and entire wheat bread and pasta are instances of entire grains.

14.Turmeric Might Diminish Cancer Hazard.
This orange-hued flavor, a staple in Indian curries, contains a fixing called curcumin (not equivalent to cumin) that might help lessen disease risk. As per the American Disease Society, curcumin can repress a few sorts of malignant growth cells in lab studies and slow the spread of malignant growth or psychologist growths in certain creatures. This malignant growth battling food is not difficult to track down in supermarkets, and you can involve it in different recipes on your enemy of disease diet.

15.Add Verdant Green Vegetables to Your Enemy of Cancer Diet.

Verdant green vegetables like spinach and lettuce are great wellsprings of the cancer-prevention agents beta-carotene and lutein. You'll likewise find these supplements in vegetables that are all the more customarily eaten cooked, similar to collard greens, mustard greens, and kale. As per the American Organization for Disease Exploration, some lab investigations have discovered that synthetic compounds in these disease-battling food sources might restrict the development of certain sorts of malignant growth cells.

16.Grapes Keep Disease From Starting or Spreading.
The skin of red grapes is an especially rich wellspring of a cell reinforcement called resveratrol. Grape juice and red wine additionally contain this cancer-prevention agent. As per the Public Malignant growth Establishment, resveratrol might help hold disease back from starting or spreading. Lab investigations have discovered that it restricts the development of numerous sorts of disease cells.

17.Cancer Battling Beans Might Diminish Your Disease Hazard.
Certain products of the soil and other plant food varieties get a lot of acknowledgment for being great wellsprings of cell reinforcements, yet beans frequently are unjustifiably avoided concerning the image. A few beans, especially pinto and red kidney beans, are exceptional wellsprings of cell reinforcements and ought to be remembered as your enemy of disease diet. Beans likewise contain fiber, which may likewise assist with diminishing your gamble of disease, as per the American Malignant Growth Society.

Chapter 5
How Sustenance Battles Disease

Outline of sustenance in disease care
Central issues.

1. Great nourishment is significant for disease patients.
2. Smart dieting propensities are significant during and after malignant growth treatment.
3. An enrolled dietitian is a significant piece of the medical services group.
4. Malignant growth and disease medicines might cause a lack of healthy sustenance.
5. Anorexia and cachexia are normal reasons for hunger in disease patients.

1. Great sustenance is significant for disease patients.
Sustenance is a cycle wherein food is taken in and involved by the body for development, to keep the body solid, and to supplant tissue. Great sustenance is significant for good well-being. A solid eating regimen incorporates food sources and fluids that have significant supplements (nutrients, minerals, protein, sugars, fat, and water) the body needs.

2. Smart dieting propensities are significant during and after cancer treatment.
An eating regimen with an emphasis on plant-based food varieties alongside normal activity will assist malignant growth patients with keeping a solid body weight, keeping up with strength, and lessening secondary effects both during and after treatment.

3. An enrolled dietitian is a significant piece of the medical care group.
An enlisted dietitian (or nutritionist) is a piece of the group of well-being experts that assist with disease treatment and recuperation. A dietitian will work with patients, their families, and the remainder of the clinical group to deal with the patient's eating regimen during and after malignant growth treatment.

Research has shown that remembering an enlisted dietitian for a patient's disease care can help the patient live longer.

4. Malignant growth and disease medicines might cause incidental effects that influence sustenance.
Sustenance issues are logical when cancers include the head, neck, throat, stomach, digestive tract, pancreas, or liver.
For some patients, the impacts of disease medicines make it hard to eat well. Malignant growth medicines that influence sustenance include:

1. Chemotherapy.

2. Chemical treatment.
3. Radiation treatment.
4. Medical procedure.
5. Immunotherapy.
6. Undifferentiated cells relocate.

Disease and malignant growth medicines might cause hunger.
Disease and malignant growth medicines might influence taste, smell, hunger, and the capacity to eat sufficient food or retain the supplements from food. This can cause unhealthiness, which is a condition brought about by an absence of key supplements. Liquor misuse and weight might build the gamble of a lack of healthy sustenance.

Lack of healthy sustenance can make the patient frail, tired, and unfit to battle contamination or finish malignant growth treatment. Accordingly, ailing health can diminish the patient's satisfaction and become hazardous. Unhealthiness might be aggravated on the off chance that the disease develops or spreads.
Eating the perfect proportion of protein and calories is significant for mending, battling contamination, and having sufficient energy.

5. Anorexia and cachexia are normal reasons for the lack of healthy sustenance in malignant growth patients.
Anorexia is the deficiency of craving or wanting to eat. It is a typical side effect in patients with malignant growth. Anorexia might happen right off the bat in the sickness or later, assuming that the malignant growth develops or spreads. A few patients as of now have anorexia when they are determined to have malignant growth. Most patients who have progressed malignant growth will have anorexia. Anorexia is the most widely recognized reason for unhealthiness in disease patients.

Cachexia is a condition set apart by shortcomings, weight reduction, and fat and muscle misfortune. Normal in patients with cancers influence eating and absorption. It can happen in disease patients who are eating great, yet are not putting away fat and muscle in light of growth development.

A few growths have an impact on how the body utilizes specific supplements. The body's utilization of protein, starches, and fat might change when cancers are in the stomach, digestive tract, or head and neck. A patient might appear to be eating enough, yet the body will be unable to ingest every one of the supplements from the food.

Malignant growth patients might have anorexia and cachexia simultaneously.

Impacts of disease treatment on nourishment.
Central issues
1. Radiation Treatment:
Radiation treatment kills cells in the therapy region.

Radiation treatment might influence sustenance.

2. Medical procedure:
The medical procedure builds the body's requirement for supplements and energy.
Medical procedures to the head, neck, throat, stomach or digestive tracts might influence sustenance.

3. Immunotherapy:
Immunotherapy might influence sustenance.

4. Foundational microorganism Relocate:
Patients who get a foundational microorganism relocation have extraordinary nourishment needs.

5. Chemotherapy and Chemical Treatment:
Chemotherapy and chemical treatment influence nourishment in various ways.

Chemotherapy influences cells generally through the body. Chemotherapy utilizes medications to stop the development of disease cells, either by killing the cells or by preventing them from partitioning. Solid cells that regularly develop and isolate rapidly may likewise be killed. These remember cells for the mouth and intestinal system.

The chemical treatment adds, blocks, or eliminates chemicals. It could be utilized to slow or stop the development of specific diseases. A few sorts of chemical treatments might cause weight gain.

Chemotherapy and chemical treatment cause different nourishment issues.
Incidental effects from chemotherapy might create issues with eating and assimilation. At the point when more than one chemotherapy drug is given, each medication might cause different aftereffects or when medications cause a similar incidental effect, the incidental effect might be more serious.

The accompanying aftereffects are normal:
1. Loss of craving.
2. Queasiness.
3. Retching.
4. Dry mouth.
5. Bruises in the mouth or throat.
6. Changes in the manner food tastes.
7. Inconvenience gulping.
8. Feeling full after eating a modest quantity of food.
9. Stoppage.
10. The runs.
11. Patients who get chemical treatment might require changes in their eating regimen to forestall weight gain.

1. Radiation Treatment
Radiation treatment kills cells in the therapy region.

Radiation treatment kills cancer cells and sound cells in the therapy region. How serious the secondary effects rely upon the accompanying:

1. The piece of the body that is dealt with.
2. The absolute portion of radiation and the way things are given.

Radiation treatment might influence sustenance.

Radiation treatment to any piece of the stomach-related framework has incidental effects that cause sustenance issues. The greater part of the secondary effects starts half a month after radiation treatment starts and disappears half a month after it is done. A few secondary effects can go on for months or years after treatment closes.

Coming up next are a portion of the more normal incidental effects:

For radiation treatment to the mind or head and neck:

1. Loss of craving.
2. Queasiness.
3. Spewing.
4. Dry mouth or thick spit. A prescription might be given to treat a dry mouth.
5. Sore mouth and gums.
6. Changes in the manner food tastes.
7. Inconvenience gulping.
8. Torment while gulping.
9. Being not able to completely open the mouth.
10. For radiation treatment to the chest
11. Loss of craving.
12. Queasiness.
13. Spewing.
14. Inconvenience gulping.
15. Torment while gulping.
16. Gagging or breathing issues brought about by changes in the upper throat.
17. For radiation treatment to the mid-region, pelvis, or rectum
18. Queasiness.
19. Spewing.
20. Entrail deterrent.
21. Colitis.
22. Looseness of the bowels.
23. Radiation treatment may likewise cause sleepiness, which can prompt a diminishing craving.

2. Medical procedure:

Medical procedure expands the body's requirement for supplements and energy.

The body needs additional energy and supplements to mend wounds, battle disease, and recuperate from a medical procedure. On the off chance that the patient is malnourished before a medical procedure, it might bring on some issues during recuperation, like unfortunate mending or contamination. For these patients, sustenance care might start before a medical procedure.

Medical procedures to the head, neck, throat, stomach or digestive tracts might influence nourishment.
Most malignant growth patients are treated with a medical procedure. A medical procedure that eliminates all or a piece of specific organs can influence a patient's capacity to eat and process food.

Coming up next are nourishment issues brought about by a medical procedure:
1. Loss of hunger.
2. Inconvenience biting.
3. Inconvenience gulping.
4. Feeling full in the wake of eating a limited quantity of food.

3. Immunotherapy:
Immunotherapy might influence nourishment.
The results of immunotherapy are different for every patient and the kind of immunotherapy drug given.

The accompanying nourishment issues are normal:
1. Sluggishness.
2. Fever.
3. Sickness.
4. Heaving.
5. Loose bowels.

4. Foundational Microorganism Relocate:
Patients who get an undifferentiated organism relocate have unique nourishment needs.
Chemotherapy, radiation treatment, and different meds utilized previously or during a foundational microorganism relocation may cause incidental effects that hold a patient back from eating and processing food not surprisingly.

Normal secondary effects incorporate the accompanying:

1. Mouth and throat bruises.
2. Looseness of the bowels.

Patients who get an undeveloped cell relocation have a high gamble of disease. Chemotherapy or radiation treatment given before the transfer declines the number of white platelets, which battle the disease. These patients actually must find out about safe food, take care and keep away from food sources that might cause contamination.

After an immature microorganism relocates, patients are in danger of intense or constant Graft-Versus-Host Disease (GVHD). GVHD might influence the gastrointestinal plot or liver and change the patient's capacity to eat or ingest supplements from food.

Central issues:
The medical care group might pose inquiries about diet and weight history.
Advising and diet changes are made to work on the patient's nourishment.
The objective of nourishment treatment for patients who have progressed disease relies upon the general arrangement of care.
The medical care group might pose inquiries about diet and weight history.
Screening is utilized to search for medical conditions that influence the gamble of unfortunate nourishment. This can take care of finding assuming the patient is probably going to become malnourished, and if nourishment treatment is required.

The medical services group might pose inquiries about the accompanying:

1. Weight changes over the last year.
2. Changes in the sum and kind of food eaten.
3. Issues that have impacted eating, like loss of craving, sickness, retching, loose bowels, blockage, mouth wounds, dry mouth, changes in taste and smell, or agony.
4. Capacity to walk and do different exercises of day-to-day living (dressing, getting into or out of a bed or seat, cleaning up or showering, and utilizing the latrine).
5. An actual test is finished to look at the body for general well-being and indications of infection. The patient is checked for indications of deficiency of weight, fat, muscle, and liquid development in the body.

Guiding and diet changes are made to work on the patient's sustenance.
An enrolled dietitian can work with patients and their families to direct them on ways of working on the patient's nourishment. The enrolled dietitian gives care in light of the patient's nourishment and diet needs. Changes to the eating routine are made to assist with diminishing side effects from disease or malignant growth treatment. These progressions might be in the sorts and measures of food, how frequently a patient eats, and how food is eaten (for instance, at a specific temperature or taken with a straw).

An enlisted dietitian works with different individuals from the medical care group to look at the patient's wholesome well-being during malignant growth therapy and recuperation. Notwithstanding the dietitian, the medical care group might incorporate the accompanying:

Doctor.
Nurse.
Social laborer.
Analyst.
The objective of nourishment treatment for patients who have progressed disease relies upon the general arrangement of care.

The objective of nourishment treatment in patients with cutting-edge disease is to provide patients with the most ideal personal satisfaction and control side effects that cause trouble.

Patients with cutting-edge malignant growth might be treated with anticancer treatment and palliative consideration, palliative consideration alone, or might be in hospice care. Sustenance objectives will be different for every patient. A few sorts of treatments might be halted on the off chance that they are not aiding the patient.

As the focal point of care goes from disease treatment to hospice or end-of-life care, nourishment objectives might turn out to be less forceful, and a chance to mind intended to keep the patient as agreeable as could be expected

Treatment of Side effects:
1. Central issues
2. Anorexia
3. Queasiness
4. Spewing
5. Dry Mouth
6. Mouth Injuries
7. Taste Changes
8. Sore Throat and Inconvenience Gulping
9. Lactose Bigotry
10. Weight Gain

At the point when symptoms of disease or malignant growth treatment influence typical eating, changes can be made to assist the patient with getting the supplements they need. Eating food sources that are high in calories, protein, nutrients, and minerals is significant. Dinners ought to be wanted to meet the patient's nourishment needs and tastes in food.

Coming up next are a portion of the more normal side effects brought about by malignant growth and disease treatment and ways of treating or controlling them.

1. Anorexia:
The next may assist malignant growth patients who with having anorexia (loss of hunger or want to eat):

Eat food sources that are high in protein and calories.
Coming up next are high-protein food decisions:
1. Beans.
2. Chicken.
3. Fish.
4. Meat.
5. Yogurt.
6. Eggs.

Add additional protein and calories to food, for example, utilizing protein-invigorated milk.

1. Eat high-protein food sources first in your dinner when your craving is most grounded.
2. Taste just limited quantities of fluids during dinners.
3. Drink milkshakes, smoothies, squeezes, or soups if you don't want to eat strong food sources.
4. Eat food sources that smell pleasant.
5. Attempt new food sources and new recipes.
6. Attempt blenderized drinks that are high in supplements (check with your PCP or enlisted dietitian first).
7. Eat little dinners and sound snacks frequently for the day.
8. Eat bigger dinners when you feel good and are refreshed.
9. Eat your biggest feast when you feel hungriest, whether at breakfast, lunch, or supper.
10. Make and store modest quantities of the most loved food varieties so they are prepared to eat when you are ravenous.
11. Be essentially as dynamic as conceivable so you will have a decent craving.
12. Clean your teeth and wash your mouth to ease side effects and delayed flavor impressions.
13. Converse with your primary care physician or enlisted dietitian if you have eating issues like queasiness, heaving, or changes in how food varieties taste and smell.

On the off chance that these eating regimen changes don't assist with anorexia, tube feedings might be required so you will get an adequate number of supplements every day.

Prescriptions might be given to increase hunger.

2. Queasiness
The next may assist malignant growth patients with controlling sickness:

1. Pick food varieties that allure you. Try not to drive yourself to eat food that causes you to feel debilitated. Try not to eat your #1 food source, to abstain from connecting them to being wiped out.
2. Eat food sources that are dull, delicate, and simple to process, as opposed to weighty dinners.
3. Eat dry food sources, for example, wafers, breadsticks, or toast for the day.
4. Eat food varieties that are kind to your stomach, like white toast, plain yogurt, and clear stock.
5. Eat dry toast or wafers before getting up if you have queasiness in the first part of the day.
6. Eat food sources and drink fluids at room temperature (not excessively hot or excessively cold).
7. Gradually taste fluids for the day.
8. Suck on hard confections, for example, peppermints or lemon drops on the off chance that your mouth has a terrible taste.
9. Avoid food and drink in serious areas of strength.
10. Eat 5 or 6 little dinners consistently rather than 3 enormous feasts.

11. Taste just modest quantities of fluid during dinners to abstain from feeling full or swelled.
12. Try not to skip feasts and tidbits. An unfilled stomach might aggravate your queasiness.
13. Flush your mouth when eating.
14. Try not to eat in a room that has cooking scents or that is extremely warm. Keep the living space at an agreeable temperature and very much ventilated.
15. Sit up or lie down with your head raised up for one hour after eating.
16. Make the best times for you to eat and drink.
17. Loosen up before every malignant growth treatment.
18. Wear garments that are free and agreeable.
19. Track when you feel queasy and why.
20. Talk with your primary care physician about utilizing anti-nausea medication.

3. Retching.
The next may assist malignant growth patients with controlling regurgitating:
1. Try not to eat or drink anything until the retching stops.
2. Drink modest quantities of clear fluids in the wake of spewing stops.
3. After you can drink clear fluids without spewing, drink fluids like stressed soups, or milkshakes, that are kind to your stomach.
4. Eat 5 or 6 little feasts consistently rather than 3 huge dinners.
5. Sit upstanding and twist forward after spewing.
6. Request that your PCP request medication forestalls or control regurgitation.

4. Dry Mouth.
The next may assist malignant growth patients with a dry mouth:

1. Eat food varieties that are not difficult to swallow.
2. Soak food with sauce, sauce, or salad dressing.
3. Eat food varieties and beverages that are extremely sweet or tart, like lemonade, to assist with making more spit.
4. Bite gum or suck on hard treats, ice pops, or ice chips.
5. Taste water for the day.
6. Drink no kind of liquor, lager, or wine.
7. Try not to eat food varieties that can hurt your mouth (like hot, sharp, pungent, hard, or crunchy food varieties).
8. Keep your lips soggy with a lip ointment.
9. Flush your mouth each 1 to 2 hours. Try not to utilize mouthwash that contains liquor.
10. Try not to utilize tobacco items and keep away from recycled smoke.
11. Get some information about utilizing fake spit or comparative items to cover, secure, and soak your mouth and throat.

5. Mouth Sores:
The accompanying can assist patients who with having mouth wounds:

1. Eat delicate food sources that are not difficult to bite, like milkshakes, fried eggs, and custards.
2. Cook food sources until delicate and delicate.
3. Cut food into little pieces. Utilize a blender or food processor to make food smooth.
4. Suck on ice chips to numb and mitigate your mouth.
5. Eat food varieties cold or at room temperature. Hot food sources can hurt your mouth.
6. Drink with a straw to move fluid past the excruciating pieces of your mouth.
7. Utilize a little spoon to assist you with taking more modest nibbles, which are simpler to bite.

Avoid the accompanying:
1. Citrus food sources, like oranges, lemons, and limes.
2. Fiery food sources.
3. Tomatoes and ketchup.
4. Pungent food varieties.
5. Crude vegetables.
6. Sharp and crunchy food varieties.
7. Drinks with liquor.
8. Try not to utilize tobacco items.
9. Visit a dental specialist something like fourteen days before beginning immunotherapy, chemotherapy, or radiation treatment to the head and neck.
10. Take a look at your mouth every day for bruises, white patches, or puffy and red regions.
11. Flush your mouth 3 to 4 times each day. Blend 1⁄4 teaspoon baking pop, 1⁄8 teaspoon salt, and 1 cup warm water for a mouthwash. Don't use mouthwash that contains liquor.
12. Try not to utilize toothpicks or other sharp articles.

6. Taste Changes.

The next may assist malignant growth patients who with having taste changes:

1. Eat poultry, fish, eggs, and cheddar rather than red meat.
2. Add flavors and sauces to food sources (marinate food sources).
3. Eat meat with something sweet, for example, cranberry sauce, jam, or fruit purée.
4. Attempt tart food sources and beverages.
5. Use sugar lemon drops, gum, or mints if there is a metallic or unpleasant desire for your mouth.
6. Utilize plastic utensils and don't drink straightforwardly from metal holders if food varieties have a metal taste.
7. Attempt to eat your #1 food variety, if you are not sickened. Attempt new food varieties while feeling your best.
8. Find non meat, high-protein recipes in a vegan or Chinese cookbook.
9. Bite food longer to permit more contact with taste buds, on the off chance that food tastes dull yet not upsetting.
10. Keep food varieties and beverages covered, drink through a straw, turn a kitchen fan on while cooking, or cook outside if scents irritate you.
11. Clean your teeth and deal with your mouth. Visit your dental specialist for tests.

7. Sore Throat and Inconvenience Gulping:
The next may assist malignant growth patients who with experiencing a sensitive throat or difficulty gulping:

1. Eat delicate food sources that are not difficult to bite and swallow, like milkshakes, fried eggs, oats, or other cooked cereals.
2. Eat food sources and beverages that are high in protein and calories.
3. Dampen food with sauce, sauces, stock, or yogurt.
4. Avoid the accompanying food sources and beverages that can consume or scratch your throat:
5. Hot food sources and beverages.
6. Fiery food varieties.
7. Food varieties and juices that are high in corrosiveness.
8. Sharp or crunchy food varieties.
9. Drinks with liquor.
10. Cook food varieties until delicate and delicate.
11. Cut food into little pieces. Utilize a blender or food processor to make food smooth.
12. Drink with a straw.
13. Eat 5 or 6 little feasts consistently rather than 3 enormous dinners.
14. Sit upstanding and twist your head somewhat forward when you eat or drink, and remain upstanding for something like 30 minutes after eating.
15. Try not to utilize tobacco.
16. Converse with your primary care physician about tube feedings if you can't eat to the point of areas of strength remaining.

8. Lactose Prejudice:
The next may assist patients who with having side effects of lactose prejudice:

1. Use sans-lactose or low-lactose milk items. Most supermarkets convey food, (for example, milk and frozen yogurt) named "lactose-free" or "low lactose."
2. Pick milk items that are low in lactose, such as hard cheeses (like cheddar) and yogurt.
3. Attempt items made with soy or rice, (for example, soy and rice milk and frozen pastries). These items don't contain lactose.
4. Keep away from just the dairy items that give you issues. Eat little parcels of dairy items, like milk, yogurt, or cheddar, if possible.
5. Attempt nondairy beverages and food varieties with calcium added.
6. Eat calcium-rich vegetables, like broccoli and greens.
7. Take lactase tablets while eating or drinking dairy items. Lactase separates lactose so it is more straightforward to process.
8. Set up your low-lactose or sans-lactose food sources.

9. Weight Gain:
The next may assist malignant growth patients with forestalling weight gain:

1. Eat a lot of fruits from the soil.
2. Eat food varieties that are high in fiber, for example, entire grain pieces of bread, oats, and pasta.
3. Pick lean meats, for example, lean hamburgers, pork cut back of excess, and poultry (like chicken or turkey) without skin.
4. Pick low-fat milk items.
5. Eat less fat (eat just limited quantities of spread, mayonnaise, pastries, and seared food sources).
6. Cook with low-fat strategies, like searing, steaming, barbecuing, or broiling.
7. Eat less salt.
8. Eat food sources that you appreciate so you feel fulfilled.
9. Eat just when hungry. Think about directing or medication assuming you eat in light of pressure, dread, or discouragement. On the off chance that you eat because you are exhausted, find exercises you appreciate.
10. Eat more modest measures of food at dinners.

10. Work out every day.
Chat with your Primary Care Physician before starting an eating regimen to shed pounds.